P9-DGT-041

A gift for _____

From _____

Requests for information should be addressed to:
Inspirio, the gift group of Zondervan
Grand Rapids, Michigan 49530
www.inspiriogifts.com

Writers/Compilers: Phyllis Ten Elshof, Sarah M. Hupp
Product Manager: Kim Zeilstra
Design Manager: Michael J. Williams
Design: Kirk DouPonce, DogEared Design
Cover photo: Corbis

Printed in China
09 10 / 5 4 3 2

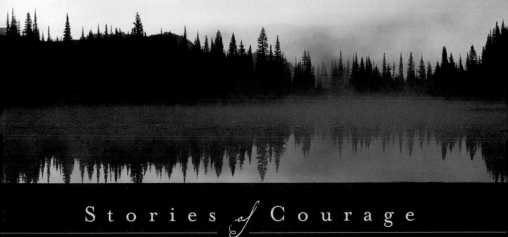

WHAT CANCER Cannot Do

Stories of Courage

inspirio®

ACKNOWLEDGMENTS

The book you hold in your hands today was born out of the strength, courage, and inspiration from many people. The Inspirio staff is grateful for the opportunity to touch lives and encourage hearts with their stories.

First and foremost, we would like to thank Phyllis Ten Elshof for her huge investment in this project and for writing most of the courageous stories in this book. Even during struggles with cancer, she pushed on—knowing that God could use her stories to encourage and inspire others.

We would also like to thank Gary Eaton, Robert Klint, Tom Sawyer, and several other anonymous people who were willing to share their stories. We have been touched by their honest telling of hope and despair in facing one of life's most difficult circumstances.

Finally, we would like to thank Sarah M. Hupp for compiling, writing, and editing some of the stories that made this book complete.

Our heartfelt thanks,
Your Inspirio friends

CONTENTS

CANCER IS SO LIMITED...

It cannot cripple God's love.

It cannot shatter hope.

It cannot corrode faith.

It cannot destroy peace.

It cannot kill friendship.

It cannot shut out memories.

It cannot silence courage.

It cannot invade the soul.

It cannot steal eternal life.

It cannot conquer the spirit.

Cancer is so limited

IT CANNOT CRIPPLE
GOD'S LOVE

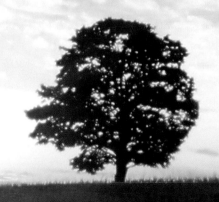

ETERNAL LOVE

*N*othing — not the probing fingers, the painful needle stabs, the interminable waiting for results, the surgery, the pathology reports, the naming of the dreaded word *cancer* — can separate us from the love of God.

For God made us, forming us in our mother's womb, knowing every part of us down to the very DNA of our cells. Yes, he knew that some of those cells would go astray, fleeing the intent for which they were created and following after their own way. He knew those aberrant cells were multiplying in us long before we sensed them.

But just as, in love, God brought us to salvation through the cleansing blood of his son, Jesus Christ, so he will, in love, save us from the truly crippling effects of cancer. For when we are most afraid, his love calms us; when we feel abandoned, he surrounds us with his presence; when we feel we have lost our way, he lights up the darkness; when we are restless with pain, he soothes us with his touch; when we lose heart, thinking we will never be well again, he restores our soul.

He does this through songs in the night and Scriptures by day; through the private prayers of friends and the corporate intercession of the church; through the expert care of doctors and compassionate hands of nurses; through the testimony of cancer survivors and the shining leadership of saints who die in the Lord. But most of all, he does this through his ever-vigilant, wholly sufficient, eternally satisfying love.

Cancer cannot cripple God's love. He loved us from the beginning, he loves us through disease, he loves us in and out of treatment, and he loves us to the end, where, someday, we will know no more tears, no more sorrow, and no more death—only the incredible wonder of his love.

FAMILY BONDS

We called my sister Jane a "scaredy cat." As a child, she feared germs, intruders, and bad food. She washed her hands till they shriveled, pulled the curtains every evening at dusk, and sniffed everything before it touched her mouth.

As an adult, her terror shifted to leaving home, traveling on trains, heavy traffic, and big cities—specifically Chicago. Nonetheless, she took on all those challenges to be with me when I was hospitalized with acute leukemia. "What's gotten into Jane?" our other sisters asked in amazement. "She's scared of everything. How did she dare do this?"

Bottom line? Jane cared more about me than her own safety. Her love transcended her fears as she packed her bags, boarded the Amtrak in Lafayette, Indiana, navigated the busy streets of Chicago, and found her way through the hospital maze to my side.

Her love also lifted me above my fears. Somehow the surgical insert of a PICC line in my upper arm to administer chemotherapy wasn't so bad with Jane's hand to grab, the side-effects of toxic drugs like Daunorubicin and Cytarabine not so debilitating as Jane fetched me hot tea, the long nights more bearable knowing Jane would be there in the morning.

Family love isn't perfect. Sometimes we siblings argue and separate. Sometimes we badmouth each other. Sometimes we just ignore each other. We get busy and life moves on. Then something like cancer threatens our lives, and we find in a new way that people who matter most are people who know us best and love us anyway. And, like God, they love us far more than we believed possible.

Family love is not limited to people with biological connections. Some of my most precious sisters and brothers are related to me in Christ. That bond is so strong that when one member of our family is struck down by illness, the rest of the family feels it as one. We reach out to each other with prayers, cards, meals, visits, and offers to help in any way possible. And because we're family, we accept the help and give God thanks for it.

Cancer cannot cripple that kind of love.

WELCOME THE DAY

friend's son, who had Down's syndrome, greeted every day the same. He'd yank open the blinds on the patio doors and announce:

"This is the day that the Lord has made; we will rejoice and be glad in it!"

Not all of us have that kind of zest for life. There are some days we'd rather dismiss from our calendars. We'd like to pull the covers over our heads and let the day pass without us. Other days we'd like to rush through, hoping for something better on the other side.

It takes something like cancer to freeze-frame us in the present. For when the dreaded news comes, we realize we no longer have the luxury of wasting time griping about piddly stuff like bad weather or boring weekends or wrinkly foreheads. All that stuff that we used to fret over becomes inconsequential when the future is in jeopardy and all we're sure we have is today.

Worrying about the future is inevitable, of course, as our lives take a detour from the ordinary into a bizarre maze of tests, surgical procedures, blood work, and treatment options. We don't know what's coming next, and that bothers us. Not knowing if we're doing the right thing also bothers us: Are we seeing the right doctor? Are we getting the best treatment for our type of cancer?

But most of all we worry about how much time we have left. What are my chances of living with this cancer—will I live to see my son graduate from college? My daughter get married? Will I be well enough to plan a vacation, finish a work project, pay off the mortgage on the house? What will my family do without me?

Psalm 90:12 tells us, "Teach us to number our days aright that we may gain a heart of wisdom." In many ways, cancer is a wake-up call that tells us we must stop worrying about a future that we cannot control and a past that is already behind us. It is a reminder to start thinking about what really matters. It is a mandate to boot ourselves out of the recliner of sorrow and self-pity, grab hold of healing, and get back to work.

It is a mandate to love each day because, no matter what it brings, God gives us *this* day and he will be with us in it.

Satisfy us in the morning with your unfailing love,
that we may sing for joy and be glad all our days.

PSALM 90:14

I trust in you, O Lord;
I say, "You are my God."
My times are in your hands.

PSALM 31:14 — 15

Do not worry about tomorrow, for tomorrow will worry about itself.
Each day has enough trouble of its own.

MATTHEW 6:34

The Joy of Work

For weeks prior to being diagnosed with leukemia, I had such low blood counts that the doctor ordered me to stay out of crowds. I couldn't go to a shopping mall, a restaurant, and most painful of all—church. What kept me sane during that time was going to work.

Work was therapeutic; it kept me on task when my mind threatened to fracture in all directions, chasing "what ifs": What if it's an autoimmune disease like lupus? What if it's a funky virus? What if it's cancer? Work kept me busy during the drag time of waiting for the doctor to call. And It allowed me to screen out the calls of well-meaning friends and family who pressed for updates.

Work also helped me transition back to health. It was a kind of turning point from the abnormal world of cancer—surgery, hospitalization, treatment, and recovery—to the normal rhythm of life: getting up with the alarm, hitting the treadmill, breakfast, devotions, then off to work.

God designed us to work, whether it's in a business suit, sweatpants, uniform, or jeans. Long before sin entered Paradise,

God took Adam "and put him in the Garden of Eden to work it and take care of it." Tending God's good creation—work—was a part of the perfect order of things.

Sure, sin took its toll on work; after the Fall, work became "painful toil." As a result, work doesn't always feel like Paradise to us. Sometimes it feels like an avalanche of unfinished projects, a tightrope of interpersonal conflict, or a murky cloud of expectations. But if it's truly the work that God has called us to do, then he will help us do it. And we will find goodness and fulfillment in it.

A man can do nothing better than to eat and drink and find satisfaction in his work. This, too, I see, is from the hand of God.

ECCLESIASTES 2:24

IT CANNOT SHATTER HOPE

Finding a Doctor

Three months after treatment, my lymphoma recurred. While agonizing over this with Ed, a fellow non-Hodgkin's survivor, he said, "You really ought to see my doctor at Northwestern."

"Maybe I'll do that," I said. But privately I dismissed the suggestion as I had several times before. Why should I drive an hour into Chicago for treatment when I could get it through an oncologist less than five minutes from my house?

Still, treatment options were narrowing. So on the way home, I thought, *You really ought to pray about this*. Two days later I was at work when I had the urge to call Ed's doctor. I tried to blow it off, but the thought kept coming back. So I finally sighed, called Ed, got the contact numbers, and called the doctor.

The first time I met Dr. Leo Gordon, I knew I was in good hands. In addition to his world-renown reputation in research, testing, and teaching, this man really cared. He had plowed through a dozen years of reports, scans, and notes on me. Now he asked in-depth questions about my medical history. He did a complete physical exam, verifying lumps I had felt myself plus others that had eluded my probing fingers. Then he connected the dots in my complicated case and made recommendations for further treatment.

Remember the little slave girl who cared about her master, Naaman, enough to suggest a healer for his leprosy? "If only my master would see the prophet who is in Samaria! He would cure him of his leprosy," the little girl told Naaman's wife (2 Kings 5:3). Amazingly, Naaman listened to the little girl, traveled to another country to see a prophet he had never heard of, and was cured.

Doctors don't heal us, of course; only God can do that. But God can and does use physicians in this world to affect that healing. And when we ask for guidance in finding the right doctor, God may answer us through suggestions of others—like Ed, who finally nagged me into listening—and receiving—God's direction. And the God of all hope led me to a doctor who has given me hope for healing in my journey with cancer.

May the God of hope fill you with all joy
and peace as you trust in him, so that you may overflow
with hope by the power of the Holy Spirit.

ROMANS 15:13

But now, LORD, what do I look for?
My hope is in you.

PSALM 39:7

Do not be anxious about anything,
but in everything, by prayer and petition, with thanksgiving,
present your requests to God.

PHILIPPIANS 4:6

IN AN INSTANT

When I entered the hospital, folks didn't hold out much hope for me. I was so weak that my struggle from the car to the wheelchair to the examining table had drained my energy reserves. Days before, doctors had told me I had non-Hodgkin's lymphoma. They said a tumor larger than a dinner plate was wedged between my lungs, liver, kidneys, and stomach. All the oncologist could add when he saw me that day was, "We need to admit you. Immediately. Don't even go home for a toothbrush." I struggled off the examining table into a wheelchair for the short ride to the hospital room that would be my home for however long I had left.

Doctors are trained to preserve life, even when things look hopeless. So IV poles, needles, and monitors arrived in my room in quick succession. As the nurse ran an IV line, I was told what the medications and monitors would do. But her instructions were lost to me as I realized that by this time next week I could be dead. The only thing I remembered was the nurse saying she was going to give me something to help me sleep.

I drifted off with anxious thoughts. But sometime during those drowsy hours I had a vivid recollection of a vacation my sons, our puppy, and I had taken just a few weeks before. We were visiting a park with a small, shallow river running through it. I instructed my sons to join hands and told them we were going on an adventure across the river!

I grasped my youngest son's available hand and gripped the puppy's leash as we stepped into the shallow river. Water swirled around our ankles at first. But when we got to the center of the river, we hit a hole, and down we all went. The boys cried out. I was scared, too, but kept a strong hand on the leash and on my son, hollering for my boys to hold on, to stay together. After a bit of wriggling I was able to get my footing and pulled and pushed the soggy bunch of us into the shallows on the other side.

In my groggy state of slumber God gently reminded me that he had been with me when I had crossed that river that day. He had helped me find my footing. He had helped us all to safety. And I knew as surely as I knew I had cancer, God would not abandon me now. In that instant I found hope.

I woke suddenly and saw my wife standing near the bed. With a smile and a whisper I assured her everything would be okay. I didn't have a clean bill of health yet, but what I did have, cancer could not touch. I had God's assurance that he would be there, and that's all the hope I needed.

I will praise the LORD, who counsels me;
even at night my heart instructs me.
I have set the LORD always before me.
Because he is at my right hand,
I will not be shaken.

PSALM 16:7–8

In repentance and rest is your salvation,
in quietness and trust is your strength.

ISAIAH 30:15

Who of you by worrying can add a single hour to his life?
Since you cannot do this very little thing, why do you worry about the rest?

LUKE 12:25–26

You will know that I am the LORD;
those who hope in me will not be disappointed.

ISAIAH 49:23

If you devote your heart to him
and stretch out your hands to him, . . .
You will be secure, because there is hope;
you will look about you and
take your rest in safety.

JOB 11:13, 18

You know when I sit and when I rise;
you perceive my thoughts from afar.
You discern my going out and my lying down;
you are familiar with all my ways.

PSALM 139:2 — 3

Getting through Chemo

When I was diagnosed with lymphoma, I jumped at the opportunity to be treated with Rituxan; a kind of smart bomb that boosts the effectiveness of the immune system. Leaving healthy cells alone, the drug seeks out cancer cells, attaches itself to them, and detonates them. Years later, I also welcomed Zevalin, which binds radioactive isotopes to Rituxan, turning it into a kind of nuclear warhead against cancer.

I was less enthusiastic when I was diagnosed with acute leukemia and found myself hooked up to bags of drugs so lethal that nurses had to wear gloves, gowns, and glasses to tend the stuff dripping into my veins. One time my IV broke, leaving a puddle of red stuff on the floor. I had to be quarantined and my room sealed off until a sheathed crew could clean up the spill.

But I felt downright rebellious some mornings when I had to reach for little doses of chemo and put them into my mouth. I hated their debilitating side effects: nausea, headaches, mouth sores, gritty eyes, bone pain, and overwhelming fatigue. I hated how they shrouded my spirit, graying out a world I have always enjoyed in full color. I hated how they made me weepy, irritable, and impatient with people's shortcomings—especially my own.

When I wanted to toss the drugs down the disposal, though, I thought of how drugs had already beat my leukemia into remission, and how they were keeping it from roaring back. What's more, they were a kind of guard dog against recurring lymphoma. So I got two-for-one protection from a handful of pills every morning.

We don't have to like treatment in order for it to work. But we should hope that it will work for us, destroying the cancer that threatens our lives. Otherwise we'll never get through it.

People in Jesus' day didn't always like their treatment options, either. The crippled man must have screamed inside as his friends dropped him through a roof to land at the feet of Jesus. The woman with incurable bleeding was so fear-bound that she touched Jesus from the back, then disappeared into the crowd. And the man with demons begged Jesus not to cast his tormentors into a bottomless pit. Yet all made it through treatment because they trusted the One who healed them through it.

Cancer cannot shatter that kind of hope.

Wait for the LORD;
be strong and take heart
and wait for the LORD.

PSALM 27:14

My flesh and my heart may fail,
but God is the strength of my heart,
and my portion forever.

PSALM 73:26

If I'm taking a pill every morning that my doctor says will greatly reduce the chances of a recurrence, it's probably helpful if I believe that. Side effects can be nasty, so if I'm going to suffer then I had better believe the treatment is worth it.

MARY ANN, BREAST CANCER SURVIVOR

REACHING FOR REMISSION

*L*ook at this verse," my daughter, Laura, said to me, holding up her teacher's manual for vacation Bible school. "How am I supposed to teach *that* to third graders?"

She showed me Matthew 26:28 (KJV): "For this is my blood of the new testament, which is shed for many for the remission of sins." *Testament* wasn't a problem, she said; it was *remission* that seemed too hard for young minds to grasp.

Remission is also difficult for people with cancer to grasp. In the biblical sense, "remission of sins" means "forgiveness of sins." It means that through the blood of Christ, full payment has been made for our sins. That doesn't mean we'll never have to struggle with sin again. As long as we live here on earth, our new, pardoned selves will battle against our old, flesh-bound natures.

Likewise, the most that many of us with cancer can hope for is remission. Medically that means through surgery, chemotherapy, radiation—whatever—our cancer will be knocked back so far that no trace of the disease can be detected.

But remission does not mean lifetime freedom from cancer. We will be fighting cancer for a very long time—if not physically, then emotionally. Every time we get a cold, our hip aches, we feel dizzy, and our fears whisper *cancer*, we'll have to lift up arms against the enemy.

Physically, we might have to battle cancer again, too. Years ago, doctors assumed that if you lived five years without a recurrence, you were cured of cancer. That's no longer true of many cancers. A friend, Mary, proved that when she had a recurrence twenty years after she was "cured" of breast cancer. Another's melanoma metastasized to the brain fifteen years after a complete remission.

As my daughter says, "Cancer doesn't obey any rules."

Nonetheless, *remission* is a powerful incentive for people with cancer. It means that all we've endured to get rid of cancer has succeeded—at least for now. Maybe it'll be gone forever; maybe not. Meantime, we live from day to day in God's grace, rejoicing for the reprieve and thanking him for this healing—and the next—until one day we stand before Christ, forever cured of cancer.

The eternal God is your refuge,
and underneath are the everlasting arms.
He will drive out your enemy before you.

DEUTERONOMY 33:27

You hear, O LORD, the desire of the afflicted;
you encourage them, and you listen to their cry.

PSALM 10:17

The LORD is my strength and my shield;
my heart trusts in him, and I am helped.

PSALM 28:7

Cancer is so limited

It Cannot Corrode
Faith

VISION OF HOPE

People in the church in which I grew up didn't have visions.
So when as a young married mom I found myself at one of the
lowest points in my life and cried out to God, offering him my life
because I couldn't manage it anymore, the last thing I expected
was a vision. Nonetheless, that's what happened. Some time
between awareness and sleep, I saw Jesus.

He didn't say a word; he just looked at me. And the look of love
was so tender, so understanding, so *mine*, that it grabbed me by the
heart. I knew with absolute certainty, from that moment on, that I
was a child of God.

I thought of people in the Bible who'd had dreams or visions.
Joseph dreamed of a future time when he'd rule over his
cruel brothers. Saul had a vision of Christ that turned his life
upside down, aborting his plans to persecute Christians
and transforming him into one of their

staunchest leaders. John had a revelation, too, of God's triumph over Satan and his eternal reign with the people he loves.

But that was the Bible. Personally, I knew of no one who'd had such a revelation. So I wondered at the time why God would give me a vision. Yes, it encouraged me at a time when I needed it; yes, it assured me that Christ was my Savior; and, yes, it strengthened my faith in God.

But it did something more, too. Over the years I have come to realize that without absolute affirmation of Christ's abiding love, I would have had a terrible time getting through the rough patches that were to come.

I could not have predicted that I would have four kinds of cancer in the coming years; I might have lost heart had I known. But God led me, strengthening me as I learned to walk with him and proving to me many times how he would go with me, nourishing and sustaining me. So when the evil days of cancer did come upon me, I could reach for Christ, knowing that he would carry me through.

While I am thankful for it, we don't need a vision to assure us of
Christ's redeeming love for us. What Jesus said to his disciples in
Matthew 28:20 applies to us today as well: "Surely I am with you
always, to the very end of the age." We who trust in Jesus will find
him with us no matter where we go or what problems we face.
We have his Word on that.

> *Unless the LORD had given me help,*
> *I would soon have dwelt in the silence of death.*
> *When I said, "My foot is slipping,"*
> *your love, O LORD, supported me.*
> *When anxiety was great within me,*
> *your consolation brought joy to my soul.*
>
> PSALM 94:17 – 19

> *Who shall separate us from the love of Christ?*
> *Shall trouble or hardship or persecution or famine or nakedness*
> *or danger or sword? . . . No, in all these things*
> *we are more than conquerors through him who loved us.*
>
> ROMANS 8:35, 37

DRIVEN DEEPER

It always seemed to me that my wife had more faith than I did. She went to Bible studies whenever she wasn't working. She never missed a church service. Then she'd come home bubbling about something the pastor had said, something she'd just learned, or something she had never seen in the pages of Scripture before. Many times I'd just look at her, not knowing what to say or how to respond.

Then the doctor said I had cancer. Not "maybe" or "possibly" or "let's run some tests to make sure," but a definitive pronouncement. That six-letter word slammed into me like a bullet. And there I was again, not knowing what to say or how to respond.

Armed with the doctor's diagnosis, my wife rushed to her Bible studies, hurried to our church, called her best buddies and asked anyone who would listen to pray for me, for my cancer, for my doctors, for wisdom, for strength, for peace. It seemed she buried herself in her faith.

I, on the other hand, retreated to the garage, to the smell of oil and gasoline, to the noise of power tools and heavy equipment.

The garden tractor roared to life and I wheeled out onto the lawn, alone with my thoughts. The vast blue sky overhead was dotted with cotton candy clouds. The grass beneath the mower was tinged with more shades of greens and browns than I could count. The leaves on the trees rustled in response to a light breeze. And I asked aloud a simple question, "Where are you?"

There were no lightning bolts; no deep bass voice thundering out a response. But I did have a sense of something. No—a sense of Someone. And then a recollection—a line from a sermon I'd heard somewhere—"God will meet you where you are." I vaguely remembered that the preacher had quoted a Bible verse to prove his point, a verse with the words, "God has said, 'Never will I leave you; never will I forsake you'" (Hebrews 13:5).

Was that really true? Was God there to meet me in my backyard amid the swirling confusion of a doctor's diagnosis? Somehow I just knew the answer. God was there . . . right where he had been all along . . . right there with me. And he was ready to meet me in my small understanding of faith, right where I was.

I still have trouble knowing how to respond to my wife's faith insights. But because of a simple question uttered from the back of a tractor, my faith is stronger. Cancer has not torn my faith apart. Rather, the disease that has begun to ravage my body has driven me deeper into God's Word, deeper into his strong arms, and deeper into faith. I can face whatever will come knowing God is always willing to meet me right where I am.

> *Be strong and courageous.*
> *Do not be afraid or terrified because of them,*
> *for the LORD your God goes with you;*
> *he will never leave you nor forsake you.*

> DEUTERONOMY 31:6

> *Do not fear, for I am with you; do not be dismayed,*
> *for I am your God. I will strengthen you and help you;*
> *I will uphold you with my righteous right hand.*

> ISAIAH 41:10

DOWN TO OUR HAIR

Two weeks from the day I had my first infusion of chemo, my hair fell out. I had been warned, of course. But secretly I cherished the hope that my thick locks would defy the statistics, clinging to my scalp despite the red stuff dripping into my veins.

A volunteer barber at the hospital had suggested that if I shampooed less often and used a wide-toothed comb, I would keep my hair. I tried both. But when I began shedding like an unkempt dog all over my pajamas, pillows, and bathroom floor, I recognized the inevitable. I called a friend from work who suggested clipping my hair back to two inches so that going bald would be less traumatic. She came to my hospital room and began buzzing.

The snappy do lasted about two days. One morning in the shower, I watched in horror as water washed off shampoo and clumps of hair that gathered around my feet. When I looked in the mirror, all I saw were stray wisps and a shiny scalp. I was undeniably, irrefutably bald. And there wasn't a thing I could do about it.

Samson woke up one morning minus his hair and his strength and all sense of control. Perhaps we feel a bit like that as well when we first confront our naked scalps. We can't trust our bodies anymore, we can't trust our strength. We can't even trust hair to grow on our head.

But we can trust God. Because no matter what happens to us, God, the creator and ruler of the universe, the one who made the great creatures of the deep and flung stars all over the heavens, is in control. He controls the tides of the oceans and the wind in the trees. He controls the tiny little birds that ride the colors of dawn.

We need not be afraid of what is happening to us because God is in control. He is so in control that, as Luke 12:7 tells us, he counts the very hairs of our head. Imagine that! Every hair that washes down the drain the morning you go bald has God's number on it. Every wisp that straggles upward from your scalp after treatment ends has God's number on it.

If God cares that much about the hair on your head, you can trust that he cares for you. And nothing—not even cancer—can separate you from his loving control.

Guard my life and rescue me;

let me not be put to shame,

for I take refuge in you.

May integrity and uprightness protect me,

because my hope is in you.

PSALM 25:20 – 21

All men are like grass,

and all their glory is like the flowers of the field.

The grass withers and the flowers fall,

but the word of our God stands forever.

ISAIAH 40:6, 8

He watches us with fatherly care, keeping all creatures
under his control, so that not one of the hairs on our
heads (for they are numbered) nor even a little bird can
fall to the ground without the will of our Father.

THE BELGIC CONFESSION, ARTICLE 13

Doubt not His grace because of thy tribulation, but believe that He loveth thee as much in seasons of trouble as in times of happiness.

CHARLES SPURGEON

The art of living lies less in eliminating our troubles than in growing with them.

BERNARD M. BARUCH

I have held many things in my hands, and I have lost them all; but whatever I have placed in God's hands, that I still possess.

MARTIN LUTHER

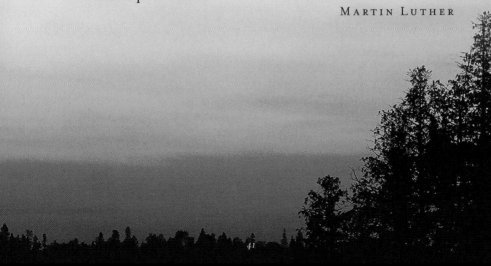

ANOTHER FINISH LINE

I used to keep a log of chemo treatments, complete with blood test results and side effects. It was a handy little reference tool, especially when the doctor wanted to delay a treatment because my white count was too low. "It was lower three months ago and you gave me the treatment!" I said, after consulting my chart. He checked his records and okayed the chemo.

But the most beneficial aspect of the chart was its visual assurance of how I was progressing toward the finish line. "I'm a third of the way through treatment," I'd say. Soon it was half-way, then three-quarters. Then I was sprinting through the final session.

Well, not exactly sprinting. Dragging, was more like it. I was so wiped out that I could fall asleep while eating supper. I could barely make it through a workday on eight hours of sleep a night, so I'd crash on the weekends, refueling on ten- to twelve-hour stretches of snooze.

Mary Lou, who had breast cancer before I did, smiled when I asked her how long it would take to recover. "Double the time you had chemo; that's how long it will be before you feel completely healthy again," she said.

That advice was oddly comforting. It took the pressure off trying to force recovery in too brief a time. It also allowed me to slow down a little to enjoy signs of returning health, like incisions that began fading from red to pink, having more energy left at the end of the day, finding food appetizing again, enjoying a morning run.

When we get sick, our bodies yearn to return to health. So when we give them rest, fluids, good food, exercise, regular checkups, and plenty of spiritual nourishment, we can trust God to renew our strength, as he promises in Isaiah 40:31.

We can have faith that one day cancer will be behind us and we will be healthy again—if not here, then in the life to come.

*"I will restore you to health
and heal your wounds,"* declares the Lord.

JEREMIAH 30:17

*Those who hope in the Lord
will renew their strength.
They will soar on wings like eagles;
they will run and not grow weary,
they will walk and not be faint.*

ISAIAH 40:31

*A cheerful look brings joy to the heart,
and good news gives health to the bones.*

PROVERBS 15:30

Cancer is so limited

IT CANNOT DESTROY
PEACE

My God Is Able

*T*his computer cheats!" my married daughter whined as she played a game of solitaire. "Did you hear me, Dad?" she moaned again. "I said this computer cheats!"

I looked at her knowingly. I, too, had often been frustrated by the computer solitaire game. Sometimes it did seem that the computer was cheating. Just when you needed a certain card, something else would be dealt.

But it wasn't only computer solitaire that frustrated me. My PSA numbers were hovering between seven and eight. My doctors said my cancer was a stage T4. They had found new tumors in my bladder. Small, encapsulated ones, thank goodness, but the cancer was no longer confined to the prostate. We had already tried radiation pellets. I had had surgery. Chemo loomed on the horizon. Where would all of this end?

It was late. My daughter gave up on her computer game, kissed me on the head, and reminded me of our appointment with the urologist in the morning. The remnants of her resigned solitaire game glowed in my direction.

I decided to finish her game before shutting the computer down. Having worked with computers I knew that programmers write lines of code to make software behave the way it does. As I played red on black, black on red, and dealt new hands with the click of the mouse I was struck with the similarity between computer solitaire and life. In a computer solitaire game, seemingly random acts are not really random. They are programmed to be there. Someone greater than the game put the whole process into motion. In the same way, seemingly random acts or situations in life are not really random either. According to God's Word, someone greater than ourselves is in control of everything that happens. Matthew's gospel records the words of Jesus assuring us that not even one sparrow "will fall to the ground apart from the will of your Father" (Matthew 10:29).

I lost that first game of solitaire, but quickly dealt another one. It seemed that as I played, the frustrations that had dogged me for days fell away and were replaced with peace. And not just a peace that comes from relaxing while playing a game. This was deeper. A peaceful sense that the God of creation, the God who is Lord of heaven and earth, the God who knows how many hairs are left on my balding head, *my* God is able "to do immeasurably more than all we ask or imagine" (Ephesians 3:20). That thought drove God's peace down deep into my spirit.

Do I have cancer? Yes. But I also have peace knowing that God is in control of everything that comes my way. Bring on the chemo. Line up the surgeons. I am at peace, for my God is able.

> *The LORD will keep you from all harm —*
> *he will watch over your life;*
> *the LORD will watch over your coming and going*
> *both now and forevermore.*
>
> PSALM 121:7 — 8

> *You will keep in perfect peace*
> *him whose mind is steadfast,*
> *because he trusts in you.*
>
> ISAIAH 26:3

FACING SURGERY

Facing surgery can be terrifying. Images begin cluttering your mind. You're going under the knife—what if the surgeon who wields it had a bad night and isn't fully up to the task? You'll be totally paralyzed under anesthetic—or will you? What if you wake up in the middle of the operation? What if you never wake up?

The pre-surgical consult doesn't help, either. Though doctors and nurses try to assure you that none of these complications will happen to you, their litany of surgical risks invites your mind to scramble down trails of terror.

Then, too, there's the unsettling ritual of checking in the day of the surgery: taking off everything that's familiar, including glasses, rings, and watch; dumping them into a plastic bag branded with the name of the hospital; and donning a faded green garment with ties in the back.

You and your spouse read a psalm together as you wait for the gurney that will take you into the operating room. "I love the Lord, for he heard my voice; he heard my cry for mercy. Because he

turned his ear to me, I will call on him as long as I live ..."
(Psalm 116:1–2). You pray together. Then the pastor arrives.
He opens his Bible to read—the same psalm that you've just read!
Clearly the words are a custom fit for you.

For someone who has fasted at least twelve hours before surgery,
hasn't had a sip of water for hours, hasn't slept well since the
doctor reported the biopsy results, and who can't help role-
playing what may happen in surgery, the words of Scripture are
a feast. They're the bread of life and living water and balm in
Gilead, and all those other metaphors we've read in the Bible for
so many years but have just now come alive to us. They are Christ
to us, calming our restlessness and giving us peace.

The best preparation for surgery isn't bodily fitness, but soul
fitness. When we have the peace of God, which passes all
understanding, we can face any operation with confidence.

BATTLING INSOMNIA

There is nothing longer than a night of insomnia. You fall exhausted into sleep, then wake up and chase the clock around the dial. It's too early to get up—the darkness of the room hasn't lifted at all, but you're tired of turning round and round in bed—and deep breathing and other relaxation exercises aren't working. You could take a pill, but then you'd be wiped out for the day.

Into the wasteland of exhaustion creep restless thoughts: anxiety about a work project, guilt about not having sent someone a card, fears about an upcoming appointment with the doctor. You know the intensity of those reactions is distorted, but when you're weary to the bone, everything seems out of control. You feel assaulted by the devil himself.

Insomnia often comes with cancer. Long nights of interrupted sleep may start after you find out you have the disease, be exacerbated by surgery, and be intensified by ongoing chemotherapy. Once you have insomnia, it can feed on itself, turning every night into an endurance trial.

A sleep specialist can help. Mine offered suggestions such as cutting back on caffeine, restricting fluids after supper, going to bed and getting up at the same time every day, and avoiding anything stimulating for an hour before bed. But what really helped me was her assurance that my sleep problem would ease once I was done with chemotherapy.

Knowing the problem was temporary helped me view sleeplessness a new way. Rather than fighting it, I began entrusting the time to God. Into the quiet darkness came the names of individuals to pray for, situations to sort through, hymns of praise, verses of Scripture. In time, I even learned another dimension of Jesus' promise: "Come to me all you who are weary and burdened, and I will give you rest" (Matthew 11:28).

Resting in Christ is better than sleep. It offers you the kind of peace that transcends understanding (Philippians 4:7) and makes even the darkest, longest night brighten with the presence of God.

By day the Lord directs his love,
at night his song is with me —
a prayer to the God of my life.

PSALM 42:8

Weeping may remain for a night,
but rejoicing comes in the morning.

PSALM 30:5

Jesus said, "Come to me, all you who are weary and burdened,
and I will give you rest. Take my yoke upon you and learn from me, for I am
gentle and humble in heart, and you will find rest for your souls."

MATTHEW 11:28 – 29

There is no cry so good as that which comes from the bottom of the mountains; no prayer half so hearty as that which comes up from the depths of the soul, through deep trials and afflictions. For they bring us to God, and we are happier; for nearness to God is happiness.

CHARLES SPURGEON

REST AND RECOVERY

*T*oday, hospitals are for really sick people. As soon as you're out of crisis you're in a wheelchair and out the door. You're still dangling drains that need to be tended every few hours, you have to stop at the local pharmacy to fill prescriptions for pain killers, and you need help getting out of the car and into the house. When you get inside, you collapse into a recliner and pull up the afghan.

Sitting still for long stretches of time is a trial when you're feeling good. We're up with the alarm to take a morning run, and rushing through shower and breakfast so we can be out the door on time. Then we're snaking through traffic to work, where we hang up our jacket, turn on the computer, check into voice mail, and take instructions from our DayTimer. The days pass in a blur.

When recovering from cancer surgery or treatment, however, we have to rest. Rest is essential for the body to repair itself. It's also a great time to feed our souls.

Some of my best times with God were during the days following surgery, when I spent long hours reading Scripture, journaling, talking to friends, taking walks, and praying. I had nowhere to go, no one I had to see, nothing that had to be done. Life was on hold. I could just bask in the lovely, wide-open spaces of healing. I was Mary instead of Martha, sitting at the feet of Jesus and soaking up his teaching instead of rushing about in the kitchen.

Unfortunately, it sometimes takes a crisis to put the brakes on our frantic rush through life. God created us all with a need for rest, for nightly repair of the cells and muscles that we have used during the day. At the very beginning of creation, God recommended that we set aside one day a week to find rest in him. So when we meet with other believers on Sunday to worship and praise God, we are refreshed and renewed for another week of work.

We can also build mini-Sabbaths into every day by setting aside an hour or two to meet with God in prayer, devotions, and Bible study. Or we can simply sit in silence before him, waiting for him to speak. If we do that, perhaps our lives won't become so frantic that it takes something like cancer to show us what really matters.

Find rest, O my soul, in God alone;
my hope comes from him.
He alone is my rock and my salvation;
he is my fortress, I will not be shaken.

PSALM 62:5 – 6

May God himself, the God of peace,
sanctify you through and through.

1 THESSALONIANS 5:23

There remains . . . a Sabbath rest for the people of God;
for anyone who enters God's rest also rests from his own work,
just as God did from his. Let us, therefore,
make every effort to enter that rest.

HEBREWS 4:9 – 11

Cancer is so limited

It Cannot Kill
Friendship

WHAT FRIENDS ARE FOR

When my friend Karen was dumped by her husband, not all of her friends understood what she was going through. Some asked pretty insensitive questions about the failing marriage. Karen didn't need people like that when her heart was breaking.

"I have found it necessary during times like these to surround myself with supportive people," she told me.

People say pretty strange things about cancer, too, like, "You don't *look* like you have cancer." (How do you respond to that?) Or "You must be very special for God to be putting you through this." (As Tevye said to God in *Fiddler on the Roof*, "Couldn't you choose someone else?") Or, "Oh, well; we're all going to die of something someday." (So just forget about the cancer, right?)

People who've just been diagnosed with cancer don't need explanations or rationalizations or even Scripturalizations— at least not initially, when minds and emotions are a thick, dark soup. We need the quiet support of someone like George, who told me months after I was diagnosed, "There are two people I pray for every day—you and Pauline" (another cancer survivor).

We need people like Mary, who told me one day when I confided that I was so weary that I couldn't focus—even on prayer: "When you're too tired or discouraged to pray, ask us to do it. That's what friends are for."

We need people like Diane and Ed and Cindy and Louie and countless other cancer survivors who are willing to walk the journey with us, comparing notes on prognosis, treatments, side effects, and questions of faith.

What's incredible is that I don't seek these people out; God sends them to me. When I feel especially needy and go looking for help, I don't always get what I need. But when I come to God first, begging for his wisdom and guidance, he provides exactly what I need. He puts flesh on those answers, sending me friends who, by God's Spirit, sense my heartaches: friends who listen without judgment when I need to vent; friends who seek me out when I have retreated in self-pity; friends who advocate for me when I'm too tired to do that for myself.

Cancer cannot kill that kind of friendship.

> *There is a friend who sticks closer than a brother.*
> PROVERBS 18:24

> *Jesus said, "I was sick and you looked after me."*
> MATTHEW 25:36

Fellow Survivor

*W*alking with cancer can be lonely. In addition to long stretches of waiting—to see the doctor, to have a bone scan, to get blood drawn—there are long nights of sleeplessness. Everyone else is zoned out, and you're pacing the dark with your thoughts. Then, too, there are those long stretches of recovery, when your world is limited to the couch or the bed.

Jesus knew loneliness, too. He traveled with twelve men for more than three years, yet most failed to grasp the point of his parables or to understand the true intent of his mission. Crowds of people asked for miracles, and bread, and other earthly things, ignoring his teaching about a heavenly kingdom. That must have made him feel lonely.

He was also challenged by the morally uptight leaders of his time, who questioned his methods of helping others. No matter that the blind had their sight restored or the lame were walking; Jesus was violating the Law by healing on the Sabbath and daring to tell people that their sins were forgiven. Surely Jesus felt lonely during those times, particularly when no one stepped forward to defend him.

WHAT CANCER CANNOT DO

He must have felt lonely praying in the Garden of Gethsemane, too, when his disciples nodded off while he struggled with his impending death. But he must have felt most lonely when God left him alone on the cross. "My God, my God, why hast thou forsaken me?" he cried out.

There is no aspect of loneliness that Jesus has not experienced, and so he truly understands everything we are suffering. He's there for us when we feel most abandoned. We reach for him, and he comes to us—in his Word, in the lyrics of a song, in a card or call that lifts our spirits. He's present in the signs of healing in our body, and every encouraging test result. He's with us in the waiting and in the dark.

And he's present in himself. As the old hymn says, "He walks with us and talks with us and tells us we are his own." We are never alone when Jesus is our Friend.

He was pierced for our transgressions,
he was crushed for our iniquities;
the punishment that brought us peace was upon him,
and by his wounds we are healed.

ISAIAH 53:5

People brought all their sick to [Jesus] and begged him to let the sick just
touch the edge of his cloak, and all who touched him were healed.

MATTHEW 14:35 – 36

Jesus said, "Surely I am with you always, to the very end of the age."

MATTHEW 28:20

If you don't already have one, get an answering machine.
Your private life is about to become everyone's reason to
reach out and touch you.

EMILY, BREAST CANCER SURVIVOR

Restored Relationship

Donna was a power teacher. She inspired me to write in high school, not just by showing how, but by telling me I had a gift and encouraging me to use it. Her support was a lifeline both in and out of college. It kept me scribbling even when I had long ceased to think of writing as a profession. Eventually, her belief in me sent me on to graduate school, where I earned a master's degree in Communications. I eventually went on to a career in writing and editing.

Still, I hadn't seen my high school teacher in forty years. After a class reunion, I finally decided to call her. She would remember me, I was sure, but how would she respond? Our intense friendship that had developed during those years in high school had been a mixed cup; it had inspired me, but it had also broken me. I wasn't sure exactly how to process that experience. So, for years I had stored it high on a closet shelf, wrapped in fear.

Cancer gives you *chutzpah*, a friend once told me. It brings you to the edge of life, then threatens to push you over a cliff. You either fall, crashing on the rocks below, or you learn to fly like an eagle. I chose to flap my wings, and with that choice came the courage to deal with unfinished business.

So one day, I called Donna.

"I've wanted to talk to you—for years!" she said. I had tea with her that afternoon. We blew the dust of the years off of our relationship, and with it, a lot of fear. And we reconciled, not as student and teacher, but as two adults with life stories to share. In the forty years since we had last seen each other, we'd each been tested by adversity (Proverbs 17:17). Through the intense heat of experiences such as cancer and personal loss, we had drawn closer to the Lord, who had refined us and now called us to work through our differences.

Rather than killing friendship, cancer can make us more appreciative of the friends we have. It can also give us the chutzpah to renew relationships with friends we haven't seen in years.

GOD'S GIFT

A few years ago you might have seen me reeling off hoses from the back of the township's volunteer fire truck. You might have glimpsed me scrambling over rooftops to nail roof shingles. Or maybe you might have caught me rolling through town on my motorcycle.

But one day I started showing up at work with bruises. I'd have to sit out at a fire with the less experienced guys because I was so tired. When I couldn't shake a cold, I finally gave in to family pressure and made an appointment to see the doctor. Maybe he could give me something to kick that cold.

The doctor gave me a kick, all right. Turns out, I didn't have a cold, I wasn't feeling the signs of getting older, and I wasn't "emotionally stressed out." Instead, the doctor rattled off a textbook name—acute myelogenous leukemia.

Leukemia? Had I heard right? People died from leukemia, didn't they? Surely the doctor was kidding. But he kept right on talking. He wasn't kidding. I had AML. I went home and told my wife.

We're church goers. I usher, shake hands, show newcomers how to find the nursery and restrooms. But that weekend when we arrived for worship, I was the one who was ushered—right into the pastor's study. A concerned group of friends gathered around me and my wife and prayed over us until a knock on the door told us it was time to start the service. I stayed behind a while, wiping my swollen, red eyes, thanking God for friends who cared.

Treatments followed. Bone biopsies. Chemo. Radiation. Then the oncologists offered something else. An allogeneic stem cell transplant would be difficult, but it offered hope. On Sunday morning I was ushered again into the pastor's study for prayer.

My friends didn't stop there, though. Someone organized a meeting at the fire hall so that folks could be tested to see if they'd be a good bone marrow donor. Another friend organized a street fair to raise funds to help us pay for the procedure. Still another asked town businesses for permission to put up coffee cans for customers' loose change.

That was five years ago. The transplant was a success, the doctors say. I'm in remission and taking medication to keep graft-versus-host-disease at bay. I still ride my motorcycle and scramble over a rooftop now and then to nail down a slipped shingle. I help out at fires, too.

But what I treasure most happens weekly when I am ushered into the pastor's study for a season of prayer with friends. Without my friends, their prayers, their faith, and their willingness to help, I couldn't have survived my leukemia, my transplant, or my years of remission. They've been more of a blessing to me than I can ever say. Truly, friends are a gift from God.

Encourage one another daily, as long as it is called Today.

HEBREWS 3:13

Two are better than one, because they have a good return for their work: If one falls down, his friend can help him up. But pity the man who falls and has no one to help him up!

ECCLESIASTES 4:9 — 10

Greater love has no one than this, that he lay down his life for his friends.

JOHN 15:13

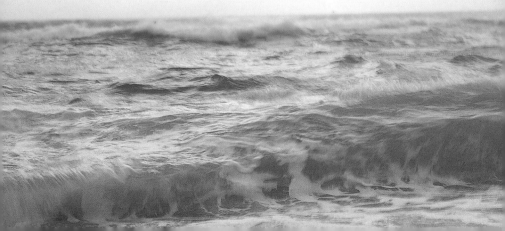

Cancer is so limited

It Cannot Shut Out Memories

THURSDAY'S MEMORIES

*T*hursdays were hard for me. On Thursday, I would begin to feel the resultant discomfort of the chemo treatment that had coursed through my veins earlier in the week.

But this Thursday was different. I had heard whispers and scurrying all morning, accompanied by a few giggles. Eventually my curiosity couldn't stand it any longer. I struggled out of bed and headed to the living room to see what was going on.

The room had been darkened, the curtains drawn, and the lights turned off. An old bed sheet had been tacked crookedly with wads of duct tape over a part of one wall. My recliner had been moved to face the bed sheet. Beside my chair sat a makeshift table loaded with blue metal disks—old, super-eight home movies!

My wife appeared carrying a dusty projector and rusty take-up reel. "Do you feel up to a walk down memory lane?" she asked as she plugged the ancient apparatus into a nearby outlet.

I smiled wanly in reply, folded myself into my recliner and slowly reached for the first film canister. Family members draped themselves all around the room as the projector began its familiar tickety-tickety-tickety sound. Voiceless images played across the bed sheet screen to the delight of my assembled family. "Look how poofy Mom's hair was then," one child observed. "And look how silly you look in a diaper," another laughed. But everyone's favorite scene showed our family playing together in a neighborhood park. As the reel unwound we watched the children scramble up a slide and swoosh down as fast as they could.

"Do it like you used to, Dad!" one of the kids urged. A chorus of voices agreed, so I freeze framed the familiar scene and ran it backwards so that it looked like the children were slipping backwards up the slide. Then I reversed the process and slowed the film so that they slid in slow motion back down the slide again. I repeated the process several times, until all of us were laughing at the simple antics of a simpler time.

As our makeshift movie time ended, I was grateful for the delightful diversion. Our old memories had turned a cancer-filled Thursday into a laughter-filled day that was now wrapped in a memory of its own.

TIMES OF HEALING

When we're going through cancer, the world can close in on us, making us believe this is all there is. We can't think beyond the disease. We're bound by it, captive to its every whim. We fret about surgery. Then, when we recover from surgery, we're obsessed with treatment. When we finish chemo or radiation, we worry about recurrence. When the cancer does recur, we start estimating our chances for survival. Even when the threat is past, we don't feel safe.

We don't just have cancer; it has us.

When that happens, maybe it's time to look back. Like the Israelites of old, who needed to be reminded of how God had brought them out of slavery and through the wilderness into the Promised Land, we need to recall times of healing in our lives.

Remember when you had the flu? You coughed till your ribs ached, your head felt like it was under a rock, and your body was on fire. The doctor wouldn't give you an antibiotic because this was a viral infection, so you just toughed it out. Eventually you got better.

Or remember when you slipped on ice in the driveway and broke your leg? You had to shuffle around for six weeks in a cast, swinging your body between crutches. Driving, going up steps, walking through a parking lot—everything was a challenge. For the first time in your life, you appreciated the parking spaces and special seats reserved for people with handicaps. Finally, though, the cast came off, and you were back to walking again.

The body has a remarkable capacity to heal. Our very cells have the memory of health. Even when assaulted by trauma or disease, they *want* to return to normal. God, who designed us this way, wants more than physical health for us; he wants us to be whole— body, mind, and spirit.

The first chapter of Romans tells us that we have, planted within our spirits, the knowledge of God. Sin, like cancer, tries to pervert that knowledge, but the farther we get from God, the more miserable we become. The only way to true healing is through God's Son, Jesus Christ. In him we find the kind of restoration for our souls and bodies that transcends all disease.

You restored me to health
and let me live.
Surely it was for my benefit
that I suffered such anguish.

ISAIAH 38:16 — 17

Through [Christ] you believe in God,
who raised him from the dead and glorified him,
and so your faith and hope are in God.

1 PETER 1:21

Humble yourselves . . . under God's mighty hand,
that he may lift you up in due time.
Cast all your anxiety on him because he cares for you.

1 PETER 5:6 — 7

WHAT PEOPLE HAVE DONE

*F*riends at church brought meals to us after I got home from nearly a month-long stay in the hospital. Homemade soup and rolls; a New Zealand Christmas feast of lamb, potatoes, fresh beans; fresh grilled salmon, rice, and a tossed salad; roast chicken, mashed potatoes, apple tarts—oh my! The memory of those meals still makes me gasp. Not only did that food tempt me into eating again; it also overwhelmed me. What generosity! What loving concern!

The cards I received were also spirit-lifters. Every day was a special occasion as I opened hand-addressed envelopes. I collected the beautiful cards and notes in a basket. Occasionally I read through them again, reflecting on how good people were to us in our time of need.

According to Ram Cnaan in *The Newer Deal: Social Work and Religion in Partnership*, it is the norm for churches in America to provide social services such as caring for the sick and needy. Believers, whose model is Christ, reach out to others because it's the right thing to do. They only wish they could do more.

Sometimes, though, it's hard to be the recipient of such largesse. How can we possibly accept such gifts without returning them in kind? How can we thank people enough for their cooking, baking, transporting, mailings, prayers, and visits?

We can send thank-you notes, of course, but that's hardly enough. We can be so nourished and strengthened by their loving concern that we're able to join them once again in church activities. When we feel stronger, we can even respond to their example by providing meals for the next person in need.

But most of all, we can remember their gifts as symbolic of what Jesus Christ has done for us. When we were lost in sin, he gave his life for us, that we might be saved. We remember that and believe. And when we reach for the cup and bread of Communion to commemorate Christ's great gift to us, we also open ourselves up to the people who are eating and drinking with us. They, too, are the body and blood of Christ, given to us by Christ to nourish and feed us.

*Let us consider how we may
spur one another on toward love and good deeds.*

HEBREWS 10:24

*Whether you eat or drink or whatever you do,
do it all for the glory of God.*

1 CORINTHIANS 10:31

*Jesus said,
"Where two or three come together in my name,
there am I with them."*

MATTHEW 18:20

UNEXPECTED KINDNESS

I once spent nearly six weeks waiting for results on an MRI that would determine whether or not my breast cancer had spread to my hip. The doctor was supposed to call, but he didn't. If I'd had a cell phone during that time, I would have hung it from my neck. In lieu of that, I stayed within earshot of the house phone, feeling like a dog inside an invisible security fence.

My daughter, who had worked as an office manager for a group of oncologists, suggested I call the orthopedic surgeon's office again. "Be nice," she said. "Don't take out your anger on the office workers. This isn't their fault."

I followed her advice and was talking to the doctor by the next day. He had been trying to contact me at the wrong number. And I had a stress fracture, not more cancer.

I pass on that advice when I hear others fret about delays in getting test results. I explain how office workers get so many reports back each day that they can hardly be expected to remember yours.

Besides, it's the doctor's job to explain those results. Verify a number where you can be contacted, and thank them for their help.

A little kindness goes a long way. In time, some office workers and other health-care providers can become your much-needed friends. I am especially grateful for two women at my local oncologist's office. They recognize my voice on the phone, sincerely inquire how I'm doing, and ask how they can help me. Then, whether it's a prescription renewal, setting up a procedure, or asking the doctor for information—they act on it quickly and efficiently. You can't thank such people enough.

I'm also grateful for a claims manager who helps me with insurance. I almost went AWOL in a paper war when I was classified as a bone marrow recipient for one type of cancer, and then developed another. Everyone was passing off payment, but the overdue notices kept coming my way. There wasn't a ceasefire till Mary took charge. This woman pursued my case with relentless skill until every bill was paid. When I sent her a note of thanks, she wrote back that I was on her list of people that she prays for every day: "family, friends, and my claimants too!"

Cancer introduces you to people you never expected to meet.
Some of them become friends for life.

Blessed are the merciful,
for they will be shown mercy.

MATTHEW 5:7

Accept one another then, just as Christ accepted you,
in order to bring praise to God.

ROMANS 15:7

Pleasant words are a honeycomb,
sweet to the soul and healing to the bones.

PROVERBS 16:24

Sympathy is two hearts tugging at one load.

ANONYMOUS

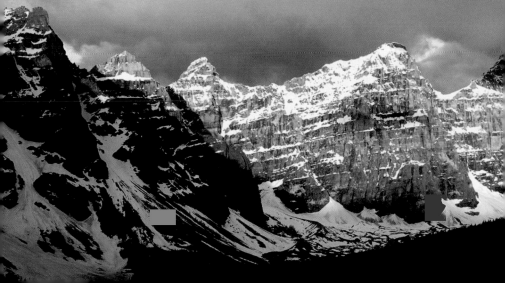

Cancer is so limited

It Cannot Silence
Courage

THE YEARLY CHECKUP

"Fear is still only an inch deep," Ellie said about her husband's yearly checkups, years after he had been cleared of lymphoma: She'd wait in knots by the phone all morning until, Howard, her husband, called, giving the official "all clear." Later, they'd both fall into each other's arms in tears, exhausted by the ordeal.

The problem with some types of cancer is that you can feel terrific and still have the disease. Other times, you may have symptoms, like a persistent cough, or pain in your belly, or fatigue—and yet have nothing more than "toe cancer." There's no such thing, of course, which is precisely the point. Eventually the symptoms go away, making you feel a bit silly about mentioning the problem to anyone, much less alerting the doctor, who orders tests that show nothing and just waste a lot of money.

Still, that yearly checkup is a challenge. It's a reminder, for one thing, of what you'd just as soon forget—a trying encounter with a deadly enemy that almost took your life. Like a war-weary veteran, you'd just as soon stuff those memories into a box and donate them to Goodwill.

This annual appointment is also a reality check, forcing you to wonder for the umpteenth time: *How safe am I, really, from recurrence?* I once saw a Canadian news documentary about breast cancer cells hiding out in tissue, just waiting for a trigger to activate them. How can we ever feel safe, once we've had cancer? How can we stop worrying?

One courage builder is realizing that for every surprise checkup, you've had many years of routine, "everything is fine" ones. Thus abnormal results are the anomaly, not the norm.

Another courage builder is choosing to view a yearly checkup as another milestone. God has brought us safely through cancer another year and will continue to carry us into the future— regardless of what the doctor may find. We can mark this as a time to thank God for healing, to renew our commitment to trust him no matter what, and to celebrate one more year on the way to glory.

PARTICIPATING IN TREATMENT

*W*e have choices," my doctor said at my last checkup.

He couldn't have said anything sweeter. After slogging through
nine months of treatment for leukemia, I couldn't do it anymore.
I was so depressed that I no longer wanted to live. Like Elijah,
I prayed, "I have had enough, Lord. Take my life." My world had
shrunk to all-or-nothing thinking. I could either do chemo
and die emotionally, or not do it and die physically. Neither was
particularly acceptable.

The word *choices* took the bars off that kind of thinking. It blew the
roof off my self-imposed prison. As the doctor sorted through the
options—discontinue treatment altogether; take only one of three
drugs; try something different—I felt hope stirring. I was no
longer a passive recipient of a medical protocol; a blank tablet on
which others would scribble prescriptions; a lump
of flesh to be infused. I was actually a walking,
talking, participating human being.

Why are choices so important? For one thing, they put the skids on a disease that has sent you thundering down the track like a runaway train. There are no stop signs, no yield signs, no beware-of-curves signs on this trip. It's just full speed ahead with you hanging on by your fingernails.

Choices move you from the back of the train to the front. If you're not in the driver's seat, at least you have the full attention of the conductor, who listens to your suggestions and makes adjustments. You feel less at the mercy of others; more in control of what happens to you.

Choices also affirm you as a participant in your treatment. If you have no say in what happens to you, resentment and anger can build inside. Rather than expressing those feelings, you turn them against yourself—or against others who try to help you. That just adds to the downward spiral of misery.

But the true empowerment of choices is knowing you can hand them over to God, trusting that he is in control of your life and will guide you and your doctor to make the right decisions. That gives you courage to participate—and rejoice—in treatment.

LIVING WITH RECURRENCE

For sixteen months I had been free of lymphoma. Rituxan, the magic bullet of non-Hodgkin's treatment, had targeted the malignant cells in my groin, chest, and abdomen, obliterating them as well as accompanying symptoms such as night sweats, itching, and fatigue. I felt terrific—until the morning I was chatting with someone at work and happened to rub the skin above my left collarbone.

More lumps.

The doctor had warned me about recurrence, saying I shouldn't get my hopes up about being cured. Still, hope, optimism, denial—whatever, kept me from looking in that direction. I felt great, therefore, I was.

When CT-scans and blood work confirmed that the lymphoma was back, I had to shift my thinking about cancer. Instead of regarding it as an opponent that needed to be dealt a one-time, knock-out punch, I had to think of it as a persistent annoyance that would have to be dealt with periodically for the rest of my life. Instead of cure, I had to think chronic disease.

In a way, that kind of thinking gives you courage to move on. Sure, you get weary of fighting this seemingly endless battle. You get tired of driving to the hospital, sticking your arm out for blood draws, waiting for bags of drugs to drip into your veins, picking up prescriptions to minimize side effects. But you get through it by the grace of God, the prayers of his people, your stubborn will to beat this thing out of your life, and the promising advances of medicine.

The apostle Paul had a chronic disease. We don't know exactly what it was—headaches, epilepsy, eye problems—but he pleaded with the Lord at least three times to take away this "messenger of Satan." God didn't do that. Instead, Paul had to learn to live with the condition, trusting that God knew what was best for him. In the apostle's weakness, he learned to lean on God's strength. What's more, God's power was made evident to others through Paul's chronic illness.

Every day we live gives us courage to take on another day. And to prove to others that God's way is best.

STEADY HANDS

*Y*ou have choices when you're dealing with cancer. You can moan and groan and no one would think the less of you because cancer and its "cures" can be painful. Or you can choose to look beyond the pains and inconveniences to find a way to help others. That takes real courage, but that's what Tom did for me.

We didn't know each other when we first met in the oncology waiting room, but Tom didn't seem to know a stranger. He'd talk to anyone. He caught my eye with a big smile and said, "Hi! I'm Tom. Is this your first chemo visit?"

I didn't really feel like talking, but there was something about Tom that made me open up. We eased into a conversation, shared our diagnoses, and then I admitted that, yes, this was my first chemo appointment. Tom grinned and said, "Well, I'm an old pro. If you want crackers or water, just ask that lady. She'll get it for you. And don't forget to ask her for lemon drops. They go down pretty good, too."

I had to smile in return. Tom's upbeat attitude was contagious, even if his liver cancer wasn't. When the nurse called my name for my treatment, Tom called out, "I'll be seeing you."

And see me he did. Our chemo appointments were scheduled for almost the same time each week, so Tom and I got to know one another. Even though he was a decade older than me, we rooted for the same high school football teams, had similar tastes in food, and had a connecting point in God, too.

The weeks went by. Unfortunately Tom's cancer wasn't responding to chemo, but his courage never faltered. One day he reminded me of the Bible story about Moses and a battle with the Amalekites. Whenever Moses held his rod up over his head, the Israelites would prevail in battle, but if Moses dropped his hands, the Amalekites started to win. Finally Aaron and Hur came alongside Moses and helped him hold his hands steady until the Israelites could fully defeat their enemy.

Tom smiled that big smile of his and said, "If we can't find courage somewhere to help lift us up, we're sunk. The best place to find courage is in God. Because the steady hand of the Lord is on us to lift us up, we can take courage."

My chemo did its job, and I've been clean and green for four years. But I still show up at the oncology unit to share a smile, a word, and hopefully a little of Tom's courage with those who are facing our common enemies of pain and the unknown. We all need encouragement, for, as Tom said, without courage and the knowledge that God's hand is on us, we're sunk. So, as for me, I take and give courage whenever I can.

Because the hand of the LORD my God was on me, I took courage.

EZRA 7:28

Strengthen the feeble hands,
steady the knees that give way; say to those with fearful hearts,
"Be strong, do not fear; your God will come."

ISAIAH 35:3 – 4

Cancer is so limited

IT CANNOT INVADE
THE SOUL

SOUL RECOGNITION

Dad lay dying in the family room. I hadn't seen him for six weeks, so Mom warned me: "He can't see you—he's blind. But he'll know you."

She was right. Though Dad's body had wasted away from the tumor that bloated his belly, though he looked more like he was ninety instead of sixty-one, though his eyesight had failed because of malnutrition, he still knew me.

"Hi Phyl," he said. "Did you have a good trip?"

He couldn't see me, and I could hardly recognize him, but we still knew each other. We could communicate soul to soul.

What is our soul, anyway? Certainly it's not what's most visible to others. I've had long hair, short hair, curly hair, and none, but my hair doesn't really define me. I've been a babysitter, bank teller, waitress, and editor, but that doesn't reveal my soul, either. What I look like, what I do, what I've accomplished—these things are a part of me, but they don't define who I really am.

My family knows more of me than most other people. They've seen me shuck bravado along with my work clothes and slump, defeated, into the nearest chair. They've walked with me out of a doctor's appointment, knowing I've turned to ice, and the meltdown will soon begin.

They're so attuned to my feelings that they can sense them by phone. "Are you okay?" my husband will ask from somewhere in Minnesota. "Do you want me to come home? How about dinner out tomorrow night?"

Still, do they really know my soul? If they did, would they be repulsed by how I vacillate between compassion and spite, tenderness and being judgemental? Would they back away from the deep dark hole in me where depression, fear, and anger swirl? Would they be shocked by what tempts me to sin, what makes me cower like a child?

Sometimes I'm blind even to my own soul. But God isn't. As Hagar, the handmaiden of Sarai, said in the desert, "You are the God who sees me" (Genesis 16:13). And he is not repulsed. Rather, he picks me up, carries me in his arms, and assures me of his saving love.

Cancer can invade my body. It can swell it, waste it, cripple it, and blind it. But, it cannot invade my soul—for it is safe with God.

> *Show me, O LORD, my life's end*
> *and the number of my days;*
> *let me know how fleeting is my life.*
> *You have made my days a mere handbreadth;*
> *the span of my years is as nothing before you.*
> *Each man's life is but a breath.*
>
> PSALM 39:4 — 5

Let him who walks in the dark, who has no light,
trust in the name of the Lord and rely on his God.

ISAIAH 50:10

The people walking in darkness
have seen a great light;
on those living in the land of the shadow of death
a light has dawned.

ISAIAH 9:2

THE WILL TO LIVE

*M*y youngest sister, Barb, had given up. Several years ago, her oldest child, Joey, had been diagnosed with a malignant brain tumor. He was still alive after surgery and radiation, but he would struggle the rest of his life with brain damage. Now, the year-old baby, Corinna, had a brain tumor eerily similar to her oldest brother's. The growth was so huge that it took up a third of her brain cavity.

As Barb waited while surgery was performed on the baby, she couldn't even hope that this time things would be different. "Don't put Corinna through what Joey went through," she pleaded with God. "Just take her."

Finally, the surgery was over. As Barb walked over to the bed where her baby lay, she dreaded what she would find. As she took Corinna's hand, however, the baby opened her eyes and said, "Mama!"

Barb wept, knowing she and her husband would do everything it took to honor their daughter's will to keep going.

The will to live is an integral part of the human spirit. It's part of our DNA, our core, our soul. Our lives are short, to be sure; some of us won't live to age seventy, or, "if by strength," age eighty (Psalm 90:10). In between, we may experience such pain and sorrow, the psalmist says, that "we finish our years with a moan" (Psalm 90:9).

Yet everything in us wants to hold on to life. We come out of cancer surgery minus a breast or kidney or several feet of intestine and are told we'll need months of radiation and/or chemotherapy that will burn our skin, erode our strength, and make our hair fall out, and we say, "Bring it on. I want to live!"

We have known suffering and pain and loss, to be sure, but we have also known the goodness of life: the delicate sky paintings of sunrise, the soft warmth of an awakening child, the sweetness of a tree-ripened peach, the aching loveliness of marital union.

More than that, we have felt the compelling love of the One
who made us, and saved us from the dark sin within us, and now
challenges us to live a new way for him. And because of that, life is
really worth the living.

Because of the Lord's great love we are not consumed,
for his compassions never fail.
They are new every morning;
great is your faithfulness.

LAMENTATIONS 3:22–23

My comfort in my suffering is this:
Your promise preserves my life.

PSALM 119:50

Jesus said, "I tell you the truth, if you have faith as small as a mustard seed,
you can say to this mountain, 'Move from here to there: and it will move.
Nothing will be impossible for you.'"

MATTHEW 17:20

TRUSTING LIKE A CHILD

Teresa said her grandma was eighty-three, but she didn't think of herself as old.

"Does she look in the mirror and wonder who that old lady is?" I quipped.

"Yes, but she doesn't *feel* old," Teresa said.

"Maybe that's because inside we still feel like children?" I asked.

"Exactly. The soul doesn't age."

We who've lived awhile know how age affects the body. As time goes by, we collect wrinkles around our lips, dark spots on our arms, bruises under our eyes, and bumps on our feet. On a perfectly nice walk, our knees give way. Our hips ache from resting too long in bed. Everything fleshy sags or jiggles.

Cancer takes its toll, too. Though outwardly we appear much the same, what's underneath our clothing tells a different tale. Wide, white scars indent the breast, the back, the belly. A slight bulge in the chest whispers of the insertion of a portable catheter. Mottled skin reflects a reaction to a chemo drug. Some of us who have lost a breast or part of a limb and have been reconstructed have learned to sit, lie down, and walk differently. We buy egg-crate liners for our mattresses to sleep better at night, slide hymnals behind our backs during church, and remind ourselves not to twist our torsos by crossing our legs.

Our souls, by contrast, remain relatively childlike. Even though outwardly we look mature and in control, inwardly we still react like we have never grown up. We still smart like a kid at a public reprimand, still sting when someone passes us up for someone else, still hope for something wildly wonderful when unwrapping a gift or opening the mailbox. Like little kids, we're still tempted to eat what we shouldn't, spend what we don't have, and try to weasel our way out of the consequences of our wrongdoing. We still lie, cheat, steal, covet, and break all of God's commandments, even after a lifetime of asking forgiveness for sin and committing our lives to Christ.

Thankfully, we're still capable of childlike trust as well. Though our bodies are frail and beaten down, our souls still cling like newborns to the promise of salvation through the blood of Jesus Christ. Time after time we stumble in our brokenness to the Savior, begging to be made whole again.

And—wonder of wonders—the Master does not turn us away. Rather, he gathers us into his arms and assures us, "Let the little children come to me, and do not hinder them, for the kingdom of God belongs to such as these" (Matthew 19:14).

Surely God is my salvation;
I will trust and not be afraid.
The LORD, the LORD is my strength and my song;
he has become my salvation.
With joy you will draw water
from the wells of salvation.

ISAIAH 12:2 — 3

The Question

I was facing cancer. He was facing bankruptcy. Every day it seemed I battled illness and the insecurity that doctors really knew what they were doing. And every day it seemed he battled unpaid bills and the anxiety born of not knowing what to do next.

We had been friends for decades, finding common ground in our studies and beliefs while in college. Now as married men with families grown and married, we stood at a crossroads called mid-life. He had never expected to be at this juncture carrying a debt load that threatened to sink everything he had worked so hard to attain. And I had never expected to arrive at this crossroad with a disease that threatened to end my life.

Our telephone conversation was awkward that day. He found it hard to talk to me, fearing his budgetary chaos was too insignificant in the face of my cancer. Yet his struggle with finances was as difficult for him right then as my fight with disease. We each held on to the lifeline of the telephone, meandering through a disjointed conversation as if we were waiting for something. And then he asked me a question.

I could tell he was almost afraid to give voice to his thoughts, fearful there might not be a real answer. Yet he asked, "So, what is faith to you right now?"

I wasn't expecting that question, but without a moment's hesitation I replied, "If you are suggesting that what is happening to my body has anything to do with how much God loves me, or whether or not I should love and trust him, well, friend, you're barking up the wrong tree!" The forcefulness of my answer shook him, but I continued. "Whatever happens to me, God has promised to be with me. My present situation has nothing to do with God's love for me or my love for him. My circumstances cannot invade my soul. My illness cannot steal my faith in God."

There was a sigh of relief on the other end of the line. He had expected platitudes and wimpy reassurances,
but he had never expected faith.
The absolute

trust and sure knowledge that God is God no matter what was a reminder to both of us of the rock-solid foundation of our faith. Our conversation continued for a few more moments, but the mention of abiding trust had worked a minor miracle in both of our lives. All the worries about the unknown, all the concerns over who was in control, all the fears about the future—everything melted away in the secure realization that in any circumstance God is the rock and strength and power that will sustain. We might never know all the how's, why's, where's, and what's of a situation, but we could certainly know the Who. Only faith in him can keep the soul safe from every harm or worry.

For a little while you may have had to suffer grief in all kinds of trials. These have come so that your faith—of greater worth than gold, which perishes even though refined by fire—may be proved genuine and may result in praise, glory and honor when Jesus Christ is revealed.

1 PETER 1:6 — 7

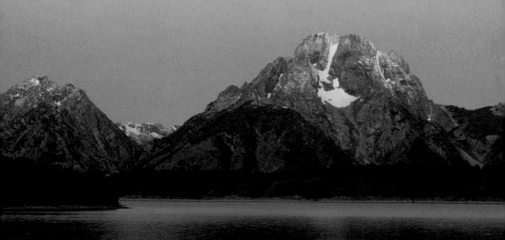

Cancer is so limited

IT CANNOT STEAL
ETERNAL LIFE

HEALING WINGS

*W*hen I finally went to the doctor, I knew the news would be bad. I'd had stomach pains, sleep disorders, and night sweats. My wife tried to lighten my mood, suggesting I was merely echoing her menopausal life changes. But we both knew this was different. When the doctor told me we were not dealing with something simple like poison ivy, I understood. This second round of cancer would change my life. But my cancer couldn't touch my eternal future. I knew that for sure.

As I child I had attended church and Sunday school. I had memorized Bible verses and knew the order of all the books of the Bible from Genesis to Revelation. But it wasn't until I heard a sermon in college that I realized there was more to faith than externals. The pastor spoke of having a relationship with God in order to have a future home with him. The promise of an eternal life of peace was intriguing enough for me to make a change in my life and recommit to more than just living a life of externals. The Bible became more than a dusty coffee table ornament, too.

When I received my first diagnosis of cancer, the Bible was my constant companion and a source of great comfort. My wife and I would read God's promises aloud before every chemo treatment or hospital procedure. It wasn't unusual that one afternoon I woke up in the hospital to find my wife standing at my bedside, reading aloud a passage from Malachi. Her hand was resting lightly on my side when she looked up at me and gasped, "You've got wings! They're all over you! You're going to be fine!"

I looked where she was pointing and noticed that my hospital gown was covered with thousands of outline drawings of birds.

"You've got wings!" she repeated. "And Malachi 4:2 says, 'For you who revere my name, the sun of righteousness will rise with healing in its wings.' I think God is telling us you're going to be okay."

God did indeed take care of that first cancer episode, so I knew he would take care of this one, too. I might, as before, "rise with healing" and go home with my wife. Or this time I might just "rise" and go home to God. But regardless, my heart is fixed on an eternal life with him, and that life cannot be altered by circumstance, even a circumstance called cancer.

BEYOND THE PAIN

Sometimes what gets me through a difficult medical procedure is thinking beyond it. When two technicians were digging for a vein to thread a tube from my arm to my heart, I projected myself ahead to when my sister and I would get back to clowning around. "We'll turn on a movie, or order lunch, or walk to the gift shop," I told myself.

That technique helped me make it through the last mile of a 25-K race: Instead of concentrating on my heaving chest and my dragging feet and the last long incline, I'd think of the long table full of orange slices and popsicles just ahead, the big hugs from family and friends, the long soak in a hot bath.

That technique also helped me through painful times in relationships. When the hurt of being betrayed and rejected by someone I loved and trusted so twisted my insides that I could barely function, I would tell myself, "We'll get through this. We'll work through this and make it to the other side."

This technique is hardly original with me. It's the essence of what people of faith have been practicing from the beginning of time. Like us, Jesus walked this earth, experiencing its joys and its sorrows. He had loving parents, though at times they failed to understand his calling. He had companions who traveled with him everywhere, listening to his teachings, yet, when their Master was in intense pain, his friends stayed away. Jesus' miraculous works of healing attracted great crowds; but the same people turned on him when he was sentenced to death on a trumped-up charge. Always, Jesus kept going by fixing his eyes on his Father, trusting him for what would come next.

Jesus died, but he rose again. What's more, he came back to tell us what no one had ever known before; that yes, indeed, there is life after death. So if we trust his word, we need not fear what is to come, for we trust that one day we will pass from this life to a place of such indescribable beauty and glory that we can only think of it now in terms of what it will not be. It's a place where there will be no need of sun, moon, or stars, for it will be filled with the light of God's presence. There will be no night there, no darkness, no creepy shadows, no cancer. There will be no death or mourning or crying or pain, for everything will be made new (Revelation 21:4−5).

In the midst of pain and suffering, do what Jesus did: think beyond it to eternity.

God will redeem my life from the grave;
he will surely take me to himself.

PSALM 49:15

But our citizenship is in heaven. And we eagerly await a Savior
from there, the Lord Jesus Christ, who, by the power that
enables him to bring everything under his control, will transform our
lowly bodies so that they will be like his glorious body.

PHILIPPIANS 3:20 – 21

In the gospel a righteousness from God
is revealed, a righteousness that is by faith
from first to last, just as it is written:
"The righteous will live by faith."

ROMANS 1:17

ASSURANCE OR PROOF

Bone cancer is no picnic. Folks have told me I'm so ornery that God needed to send a tough cancer my way just to get my attention. While that may not be true, my fight with cancer did help assure me of my eternal future with God.

My cancer treatments forced me to spend a lot of time in bed. I asked my family to move a stereo system within easy reach so I could listen to cassette tapes or CDs. Because I had many questions about God and faith, I often chose to listen to the Bible on tape.

I had been listening to tapes for several days when tests revealed my cancer was not responding to the medications as well as doctors had hoped. As a new medicine dripped through my IV, I wondered aloud if the things I had heard and read and believed in Scripture were really true. Was there a heaven? If I died, would I live with God forever? I wanted more than a pastor's promise that these things were true. I wanted proof.

I flipped on the tape player and heard the now familiar voice begin to read about John the Baptist and his followers. John was stuck in prison, but he was curious about something. So he sent his followers to Jesus with a question, "Are you the one who was to come?" (Luke 7:19).

John's followers found Jesus and asked John's question. It should have been an easy answer, a simple yes or no. But Jesus didn't give a simple reply. He said, "Go back and report to John what you have seen and heard: The blind receive sight, the lame walk, those who have leprosy are cured, the deaf hear, the dead are raised, and the good news is preached to the poor" (Luke 7:22).

I was dumbstruck. Jesus' answer to John wasn't a simple assurance, but rather verifiable proof that forced John to think. John knew the Scriptures. John knew what the signs of the Messiah would be. Jesus' answer gave John enough proof to draw his own conclusion—Jesus was the promised one.

I stopped the tape and realized God had already given me proof, too, in answer to my questions. The miracles I saw everyday— a child being born, the sun rising and setting on cue, tree leaves bursting forth from sleeping branches—all were signs of God's trustworthiness to do what he said he would do. These miracles were the verifiable proof that the things I had heard and read and believed in the Bible were true. Even if doctors were unable to control the spread of my bone cancer, even if I died, I would still have God's love and would spend eternity with him. I didn't need someone's simple assurance; I had God's proof—for that time and for all eternity.

Surely goodness and love will follow me all the days of my life,
and I will dwell in the house of the LORD forever.

PSALM 23:6

And this is the testimony: God has given us eternal life,
and this life is in his Son. He who has the Son has life; he who does not
have the Son of God does not have life.

1 JOHN 5:11–12

My Father's will is that everyone who looks
to the Son and believes in him shall have eternal life,
and I will raise him up at the last day.

JOHN 6:40

A PLACE FOR US

My husband, Paul, and I had time to kill before my room in the hospital was ready. So we ate lunch, wandered through the gift shop, flipped through magazines, watched people—and tried not to harass the clerk at the desk about when we could go upstairs.

When we finally got to my room on the fifteenth floor, we realized, in part, what had taken so long. The dark cherry shelving was polished, the bed crisp with fresh linens, the washroom stacked with supplies. There was no trace of the former occupant; this was my space. No one could see me without washing hands and pulling on gloves, masks, and gowns. I was in a sealed ward that no one could enter without first passing through a space that locked off outside air. Those inside this ward had to be protected from germs.

My room was beautiful; it overlooked the city of Chicago. By day I watched people and traffic scurry far below me. By night I watched the lights brighten the tall buildings surrounding me. Of all the hospitals I knew, this was by far the most luxurious.

I felt safe, protected, well-cared for in that room. It became a kind of Bethel for me, a place where I felt very close to the gate of heaven, and where I promised to continue my journey as long as God would be with me.

After nearly a month, I went home. That's when I realized how small and cramped that little room had been. The sky, which I could only glimpse through a window, was suddenly vibrant around me. People and cars moved past me, life-size. The world was so full of color, beauty, movement, and energy that I could hardly take it in.

I realized what a place of trial that little room had been. In it I had experienced all the predicted side effects of chemotherapy: nausea, vomiting, rashes, bleeding, hair loss, fevers, pressure headaches, infection in the fluid around my heart and brain. Now that I was home, I realized how sick I had been.

In some ways, that little room is like this world. It is all we know of home. But even now, Jesus is preparing a place for us in heaven. It's a place we don't know much about yet, but we can trust that it will be good. Jesus himself will take us there. And we will look back on this time on earth, this vale of suffering, as something we merely passed through on our way to something better.

For God so loved the world that he gave
his one and only Son, that whoever believes in him
shall not perish but have eternal life.

JOHN 3:16

Even though I walk
through the valley of the shadow of death,
I will fear no evil,
for you are with me.

PSALM 23:4

Jesus said, "If I go and prepare a place for you,
I will come back and take you to be with me
that you also may be where I am."

JOHN 14:3

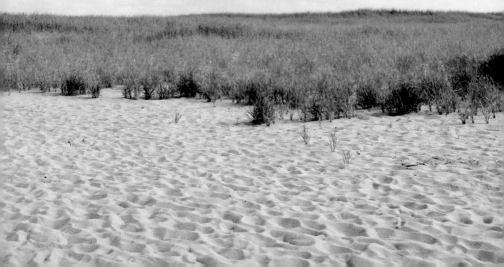

Cancer is so limited

IT CANNOT CONQUER
THE SPIRIT

BACKUP PRAYER

For weeks I had been praying for God's direction about my chemotherapy. After a six-week break from three drugs that had all but killed my will to go on living, much less my ability to fight cancer, I had agreed to begin one of the drugs again.

ATRA knocked me off my feet. I spent three days in bed with a killer headache caused by fluid buildup around the brain. I took a breather, then tried a reduced dose of the drug. More headaches—plus insomnia, depression, and fatigue. I walked into the doctor's office, feeling like a failure. I had flunked this chemo—what was next? Arsenic?

But my doc had something up the sleeve of his white coat. After listening to my litany of woe, he gave me the news. "Preliminary reports on new studies strongly suggest that people in molecular remission from APL (my type of leukemia) who went through maintenance therapy did not do significantly better than those without," he said. "I'm taking you off chemo."

I felt like life had been handed back to me.

Sometimes when we pray, we don't know what to pray for. We try asking questions, then we speculate how God might answer. Then we ask more questions with those answers in mind. But the process seems wrong. So finally we just give up trying to guess and just beg God to tell us what to do. We feel so weak and so directionless and so helpless that we can hardly pray.

Here, then, is the miracle. Romans 8:26 tells us that when we are in such a state, "the Spirit himself intercedes for us with groans that words cannot express." The Spirit prays for God's will for us when we don't have a clue what that is. And the Spirit "who searches our hearts" (v. 27) negotiates answers for us that far surpass anything we might have dreamed up on our own.

Can cancer kill our spirits? Not if it rests, even at its weakest, in the Spirit of God. For, as Paul says in verse 37: "In all these things we are more than conquerors through him who loved us."

BLAMELESS

Some of us don't need friends like Job's to beat up on us—we beat up on ourselves. When we get cancer, we wonder if it's because of something we did. Was it the water we drank? The smoking we did in college? Not enough exercise? Poor diet?

We can dig at ourselves spiritually, too. Is God punishing us for some secret sin? Is he trying to loosen our grip on things to make us more dependent on him? Is he trying to get at our spirits by humbling our bodies?

Such questions may be worth pondering—for a while. But we shouldn't get stuck in them. As my friend Donna says, "Life's too short." Cancer can prompt us to make changes in our lives, one of which should be learning to take better care of ourselves.

We could try listening to our bodies, for example, tuning in to its complaints. For example, if we have a perpetually sore shoulder, we may be sitting incorrectly, or tensing too long at the computer. A few stretching exercises could help. If we nod off mid-morning, maybe it's because we skipped breakfast. We might need a pick-up snack, like some yogurt or a granola bar.

We should take note of the times we feel especially good, too. Are we energized after a weekend of banking sleep to cover the shortages of the week, at the finish of a great bike ride, after a long walk? Maybe we should take more time for such body builders.

We also need time to tend our spirits. The Bible tells us that our bodies are God's temples (1 Corinthians 3:16). Imagine that—these faltering, scarred, broken down, diseased bodies—receptacles of the Spirit of God!

What's more, we have been washed, sanctified, and justified in the name of the Lord Jesus Christ and by the Spirit of God. That means we no longer have to lug around a load of regrets or beat ourselves up spiritually because we have cancer. We are blameless in the sight of God. As 1 Corinthians 6:19–20 says, "You are not your own; you were bought with a price. Therefore honor God with your body."

I am laid low in the dust;
preserve my life according to your word.
I recounted my ways and you answered me.

PSALM 119:25 — 26

Restore us, O LORD God Almighty;
make your face shine upon us,
that we may be saved.

PSALM 80:19

If the Son sets you free, you will be free indeed.

JOHN 8:36

But God demonstrates his own love for us in this:
While we were still sinners, Christ died for us.

ROMANS 5:8

LEARNING TO LISTEN

I'm a doer. If I'm not physically *doing* something, I don't feel useful. If I'm in a boat, I have to fish. If I'm in the yard, I have to cut the grass. If I'm in the house, I have to sweep or fix something. I'm a doer.

However, cancer forced me to put my brakes on. There were whole days when I couldn't *do* anything. I began to feel useless. But then I stumbled across the Bible story about Elijah. This ancient prophet stood his ground against wicked rulers, irritating them so much they wanted to kill him. Elijah hid in the desert, asking God to kill him instead so he wouldn't have to fight the evils around him any longer.

I could relate to Elijah's prayer. I felt that my cancer was an evil tearing me apart inside. Because I couldn't do the things I had done before, maybe it would be better for everyone if God would let me die, too.

God didn't agree with Elijah's estimation of his problem any more than he agreed with mine. Rather, God responded gently to this man who was completely beaten down by the evils of his situation. He met Elijah in the midst of his trouble, but not in a powerful wind, shuddering earthquake, or raging fire. God came to Elijah in "a gentle whisper" (I Kings 19:12).

I was struck by the quietness of God's coming because I probably would have missed the whisper. In my own life I had been expecting God to heal me with the quickness of a tornado, to shake the doctors with an earth-shattering miracle, or to burn away my disease as if it had never been there. Instead, God had chosen to let my illness teach me to listen.

I began to listen in earnest, for listening became my way of feeling useful again. I could do something. Though I couldn't push a broom or cast a line, I *could* listen. I found myself growing spiritually and emotionally stronger. What cancer had been tearing apart, God's lesson of listening began to build and strengthen. I learned to listen to my wife, to give her time to vent without trying to solve anything. I listened to my doctors, to hear what they said and how they said it so I could make better choices.

I learned to listen to my body, too, to read the signals that I had been too busy to notice before.

But most of all I learned to listen to God. Rather than just bringing a laundry list of needs to him in prayer, I now found strength in waiting for the whisper of his presence. Though cancer and its cures ravaged my body for a time, it never conquered my spirit. In learning to listen, I let God's still, small voice whisper strength to my weakness, hope to my heart, and health to my spirit.

He who forms the mountains, creates the wind, and reveals his thoughts to man, he who turns dawn to darkness, and treads the high places of the earth — the Lord God Almighty is his name.

AMOS 4:13

Praise be to the God and Father of our Lord Jesus Christ, the Father of compassion and the God of all comfort, who comforts us in all our troubles, so that we can comfort those in any trouble with the comfort we ourselves have received from God.

2 CORINTHIANS 1:3 — 4

CHOOSE JOY

When the doctor told me the mass he found was malignant, I grimaced. But then I considered that the Bible is full of reminders to "rejoice." I didn't want cancer to rob me of my true source of strength, so I bowed my spirit in prayer, dug down deep, and asked God to grant me a joyful heart.

What a difference that prayer made. My cancer would involve three unpleasant treatment protocols, including surgery, radiation, and chemotherapy. Into all of those treatment rooms, I carried God's joy. With the surgical team in pre-op, I swapped jokes. In the recovery room after surgery, I sported a weak but recognizable smile. A nurse commented to my wife that she didn't mind coming in to my room to care for me because even though I was very sick, I was always upbeat. My wife was able to tell her I wasn't a saint, but that I had prayed for God's joy.

When the radiation treatments started, I continued to focus on joy. I joked with the radiologist, asking if he were merely using my body as a practice canvas for a dot-to-dot book. I met people in the waiting room who became close friends because we shared the humor of our tough situations with each other. The smiles, encouragement and joy that God gave in all of those treatments splashed refreshingly from one to another.

My chemo treatments were the hardest protocols, yet joy remained my companion. No one truly enjoys the metallic taste of food or watching clumps of hair fall into the sink unexpectedly. But when my dog licked my chemo-bald head as it rested on the arm of the sofa, well, that made me laugh. What was that dog thinking? My head must have looked like some strange doggy treat. God answered a prayer for joy with a strange, unexpected, and truly funny, doggy slurp.

Today the doctor says the cancer is gone for now. But the lessons I learned about joy in that testing time have stayed with me. Choosing to be joyful in spite of cancer makes your spirit come alive, because you have chosen to do something that's full of life, not disease; full of hope, not pain; full of laughter, not tears. So if the cancer returns, I'll meet it with God's help—and choose joy.

At Inspirio, we would love to hear your stories and your feedback.
Please send your comments to us by way of email at
icares@zondervan.com or to the address below:

inspirio

Attn: Inspirio Cares
5300 Patterson Avenue SE
Grand Rapids, MI 49530

If you would like further information about Inspirio
and the products we create, please visit us at:
www.inspiriogifts.com

Thank you and God bless!